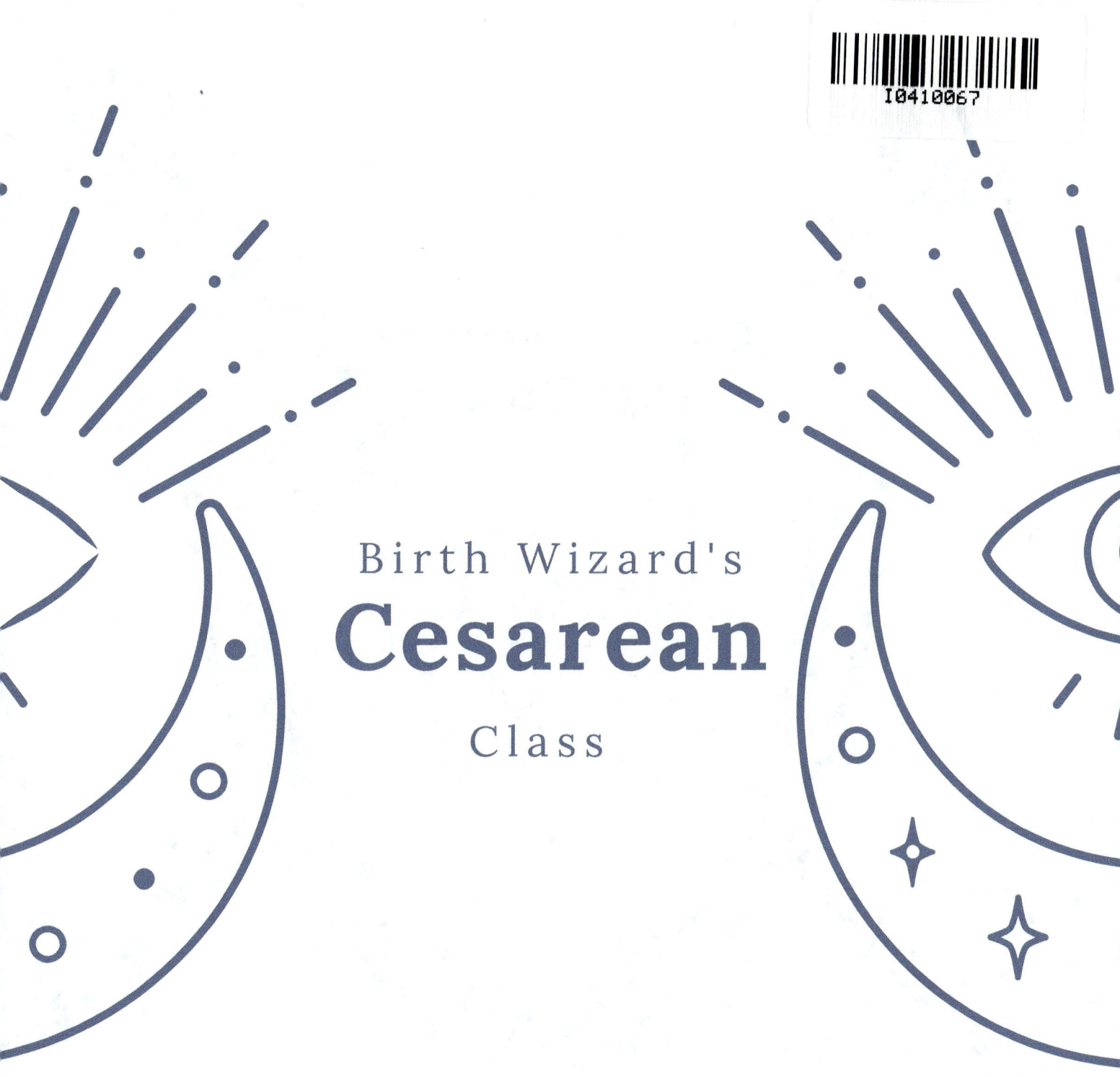

Birth Wizard's
Cesarean
Class

School of the Birth Wizardry
Tome of Birth Wisdom
Volume II: Cesarean

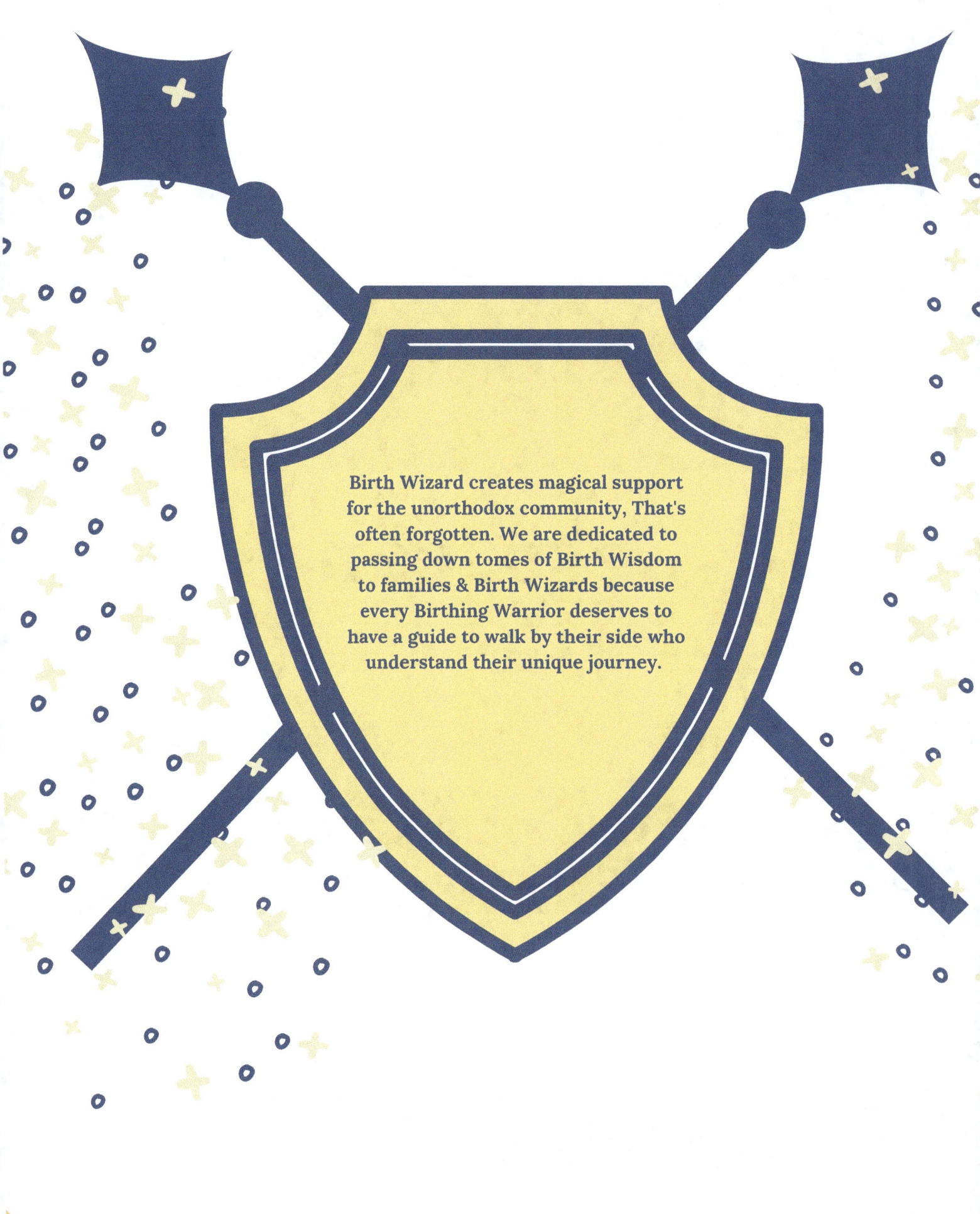

Birth Wizard creates magical support for the unorthodox community, That's often forgotten. We are dedicated to passing down tomes of Birth Wisdom to families & Birth Wizards because every Birthing Warrior deserves to have a guide to walk by their side who understand their unique journey.

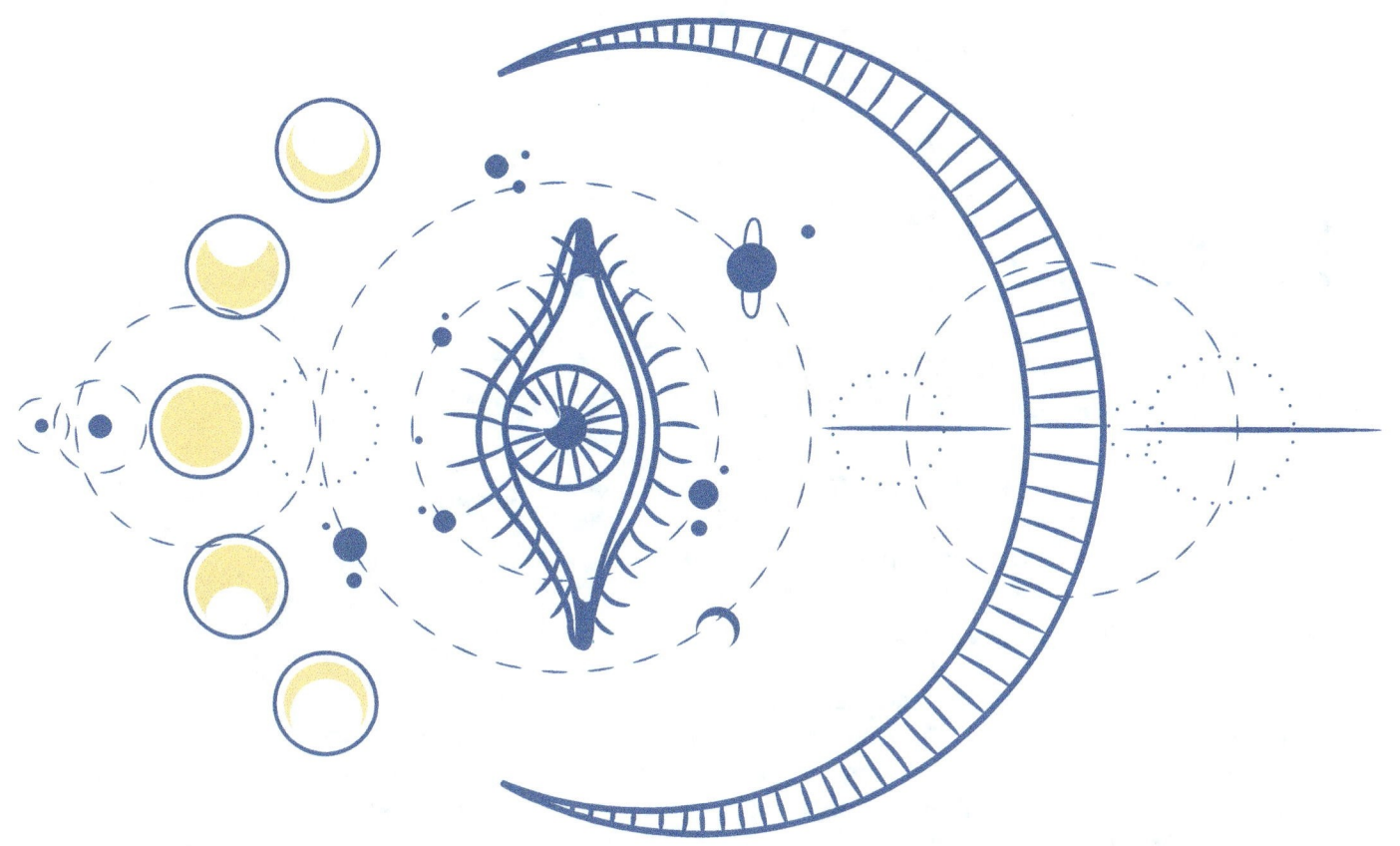

Table of Contents

Huzzah! Welcome!

I appreciate you taking this unique class to guide through your Cesarean Birth journey. This class was developed with care, understanding and knowing how important this is to you. My own quest for an empowered Birth is what led me to be an advocate, doula and educator.

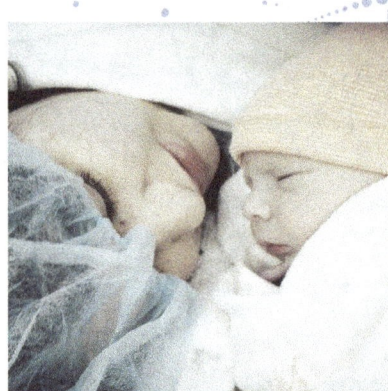

My first pregnancy "was a dream" and assumed that childbirth would be the same. I was the "perfect patient", meaning I never questioned anything the doctor's or hospital told me, and like 1 in 3 women in America, this resulted in a C-section. My cesarean birth wasn't a birth. It was a surgery.

I spent almost a year researching, joining groups, attending therapy, and reading everything I could get my hands on about vaginal birth and C-sections. I knew if I didn't achieve my VBAC, I wanted to have my empowered birth.

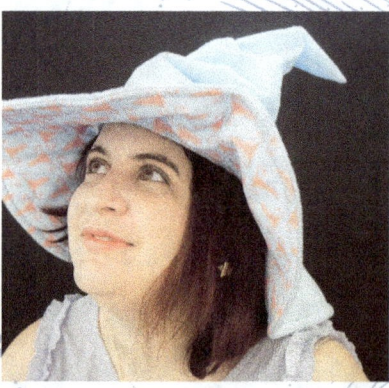

After becoming a Doula and Educator, I realized how hard it was to get support that wasn't biased or uneducated towards Cesarean Birth. I became a mentor and advocate in my community to make sure other birth workers could speak with confidence and with education about Cesarean birth. I also supported countless Birthers to have a beautiful Cesarean Birth.

Your Birth Wizard is always excited to help with any extra assistance you need on your journey. I'm always excited to hear from participants of this course. Summon any Birth Wizard by sending an email or carrier pigeon.

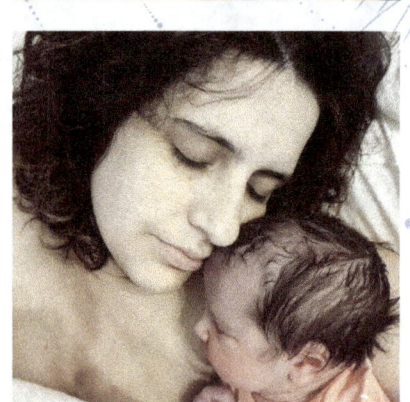

Here's to you and your future empowered birth

Emmy Howard

Ancient History

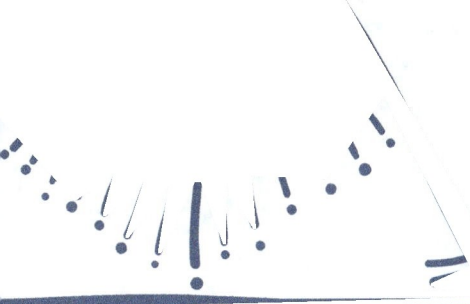

_____ clan in England introduced obstetrical forceps to pull from the birth canal fetuses in _____'s

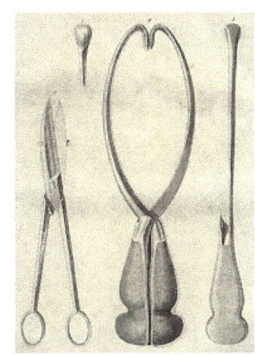

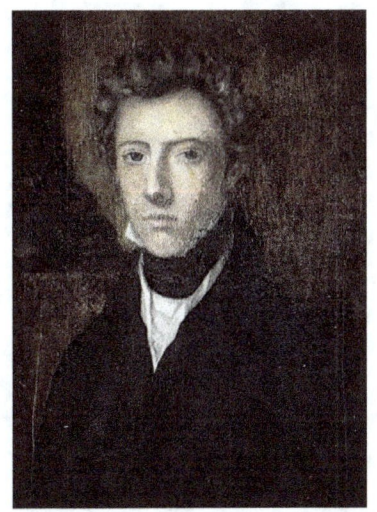

_____ _____ is famous for performing first successful cesarean birth in United Kingdom

Skills he picked up from the indigenous people of _____ Kingdom

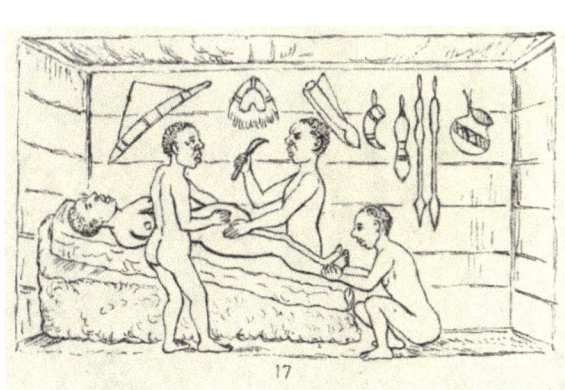

Modern History

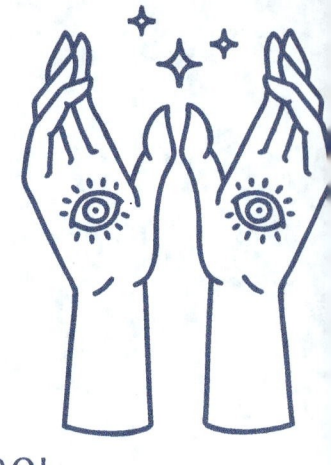

1970's

1980's

2010

2018

Preparing For Birth

```
S W H A C G B I R T H P L A N
R D G L U A I D V L H N Z F O
P P U U O B R Y V G P X R R I
W F H O P L X P N T E N P E T
R E F D V A Y I L X S Z Q E A
F J W M Z T S C X J J D N Z R
Z B C U U I T N P J H O M E A
F C P T C P L N N Z I Z V R P
N D S R W S N Z Q T Y A M M E
U E E A R O A I I N W S O E R
G X S P R H P R T A R X A A P
E R A T J P T Q A Y G Q J L D
L G C S I U W D C Z C T X S N
Z F R O N N Z Q F I D Q J E I
P U V P P Z G K R W H Q S I M
```

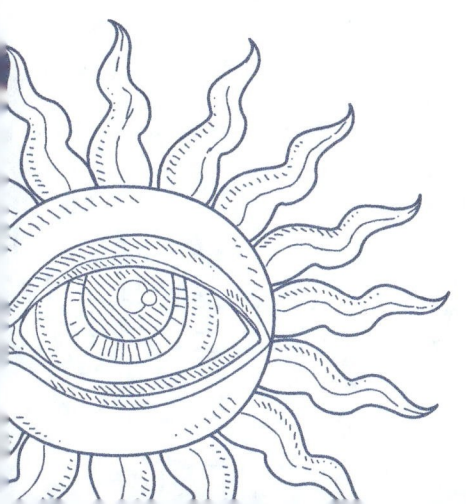

Preamble to Birth

Birth Research

Understanding every
option available to you
and how it could
impact your birth

Braxton Hicks

sporadic contractions and
relaxation of the uterine
muscle

Prodromal Labor

labor that starts and
stops before fully active
labor begins

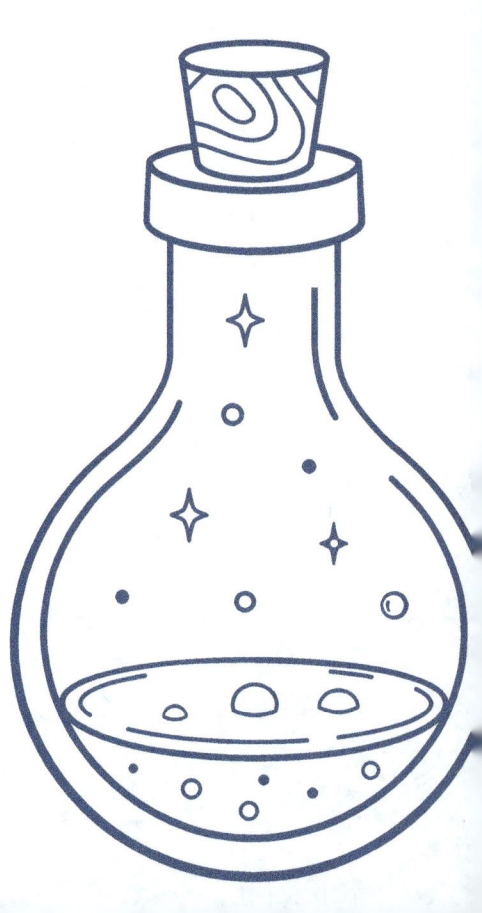

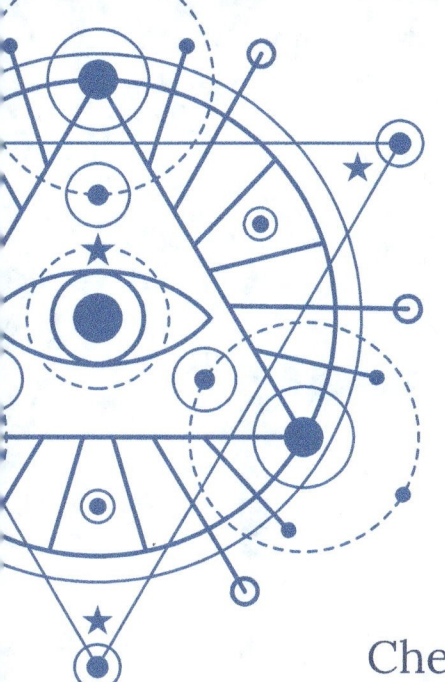

Before Birth

Checklist

- ◯ Check into Hospital 2 hours before Birth

- ◯ Pre-Op (Blood Tests, Blood Pressure, IV Fluids and ect)

- ◯ Meeting your team

- ◯ Epidural/Anastetics are placed

- ◯ Signing any forms

- ◯ Music Selected

- ◯ Partner puts on bunny outfit

- ◯ Place Wraps (SCDs) on your legs to prevent blood cots

- ◯ Wash your Abdomen

- ◯ Place of Foley Catheter

- ◯ Drink an Antacid Drink

During Birth

Rolled into room

Checklist is completed

Sterile Screen goes up

Surgery starts

Baby is born within 10 minutes

Baby exams

Common Sensations

Intense Tugging
Burning
Pressure in chest
Drowsy
Shakes
Nausea
Various Smells

Layers of Cesarean

Layer 1   Skin lower abdominal wall

Layer 2   Subcutaneous fat

Layer 3   Fascia

Layer 4   Rectus Abdominis (separated not cut)

Layer 5   Thin Transverse fascia and peritoneum

Layer 6   Bladder flap under retractor

Layer 7   Wall of lower uterine segment

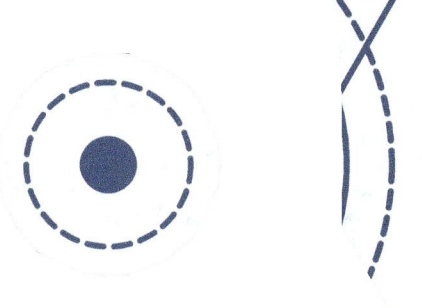

After Birth

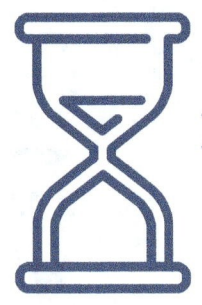

Moved to Recovery up to 2 Hours after exiting OR

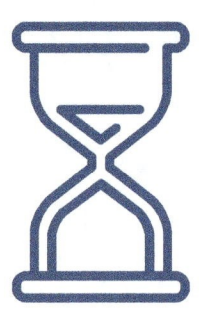

Fundus Massage

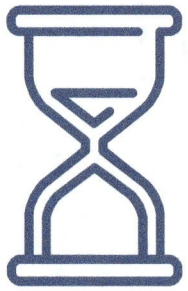

Pain Medication and Stool softeners encouraged up to 2 days after birth

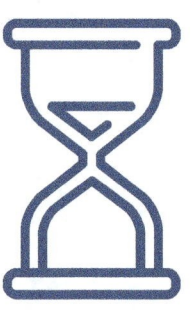

Baby can be feeding eirther through breast/chest or chosen method

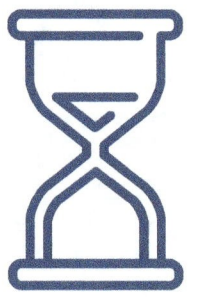

Leg compression continues until you are ready to walk

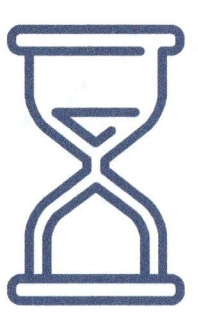

Monitoring for blood pressure continues unt all medication can moved through your system

Immediate Recovery

Things to be aware of

_____

_____

_____

_____

_____

_____

Continued Recovery

What are some of your plans for Recovery?

_____

_____

_____

_____

_____

Stages of Recovery

Stage 1
Inflammatory

_____

_____

_____

Stage 2
Proliferation

_____

_____

_____

Stage 3
Remodeling

_____

_____

_____

Mental Games

Catastrophe Game

_____

_____

_____

_____

_____

_____

_____

_____

It's not a "REAL" birth

_____

_____

_____

_____

_____

_____

_____

_____

Your own mental game
Please write the rules the game your mind loves to play

_____

_____

_____

_____

Birth Trauma

Stats say ___ birthing people will have a traumatic birth

Who is at risk?

_____ complications

Birthing Interventions

Babies needing _____ care

People with significant injuries

People with existing _____ problems

People with previous trauma and abuse People from marginalized backgrounds

NO ONE IS IMMUNE!!

___ of people try a treatment approach and it doesn't work

Write 4 resources you can use in case of emergency

_____

_____

_____

_____

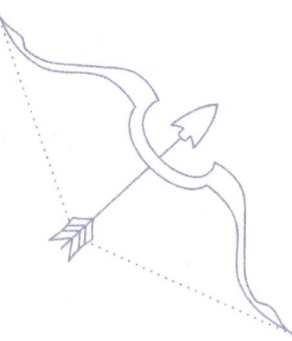

Party Members

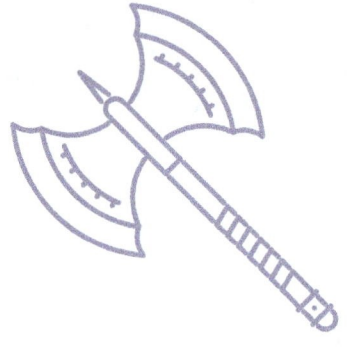

Name your qualities and skills only you
can bring to this quest

_____

_____

_____

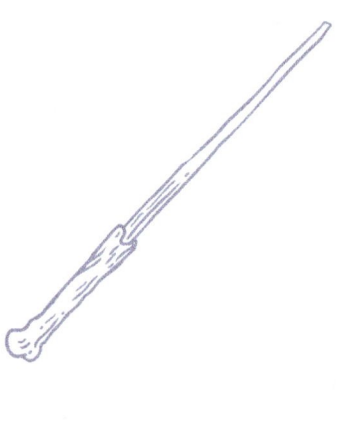

Name 3 birth wishes you hope to fulfill
during this quest

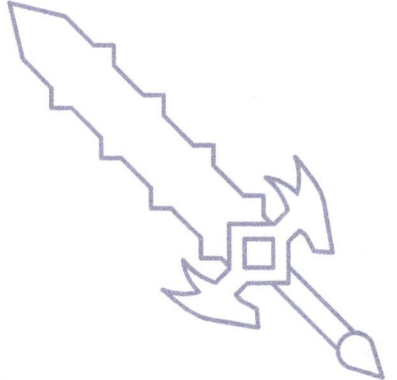

_____

_____

_____

_____

Advocating

B _____

R _____

A _____

I _____

N _____

Boundary Riffing

Write down your favorites

_____

_____

_____

_____

Fear Release

Fear Bubbles

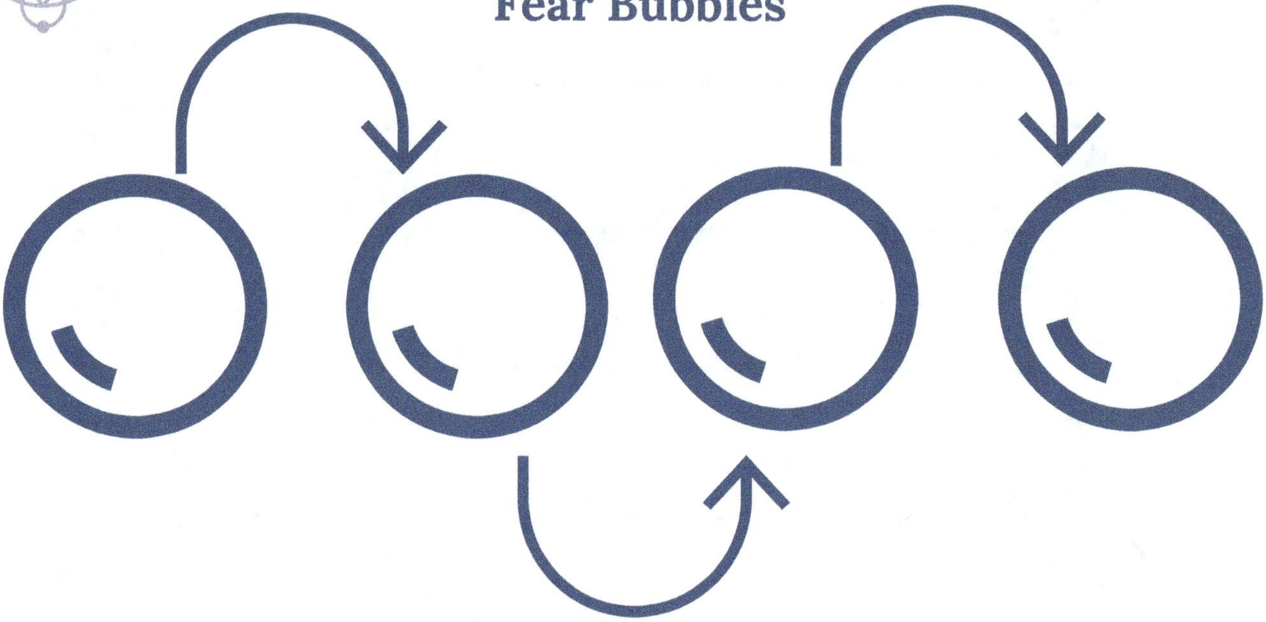

Breath Work

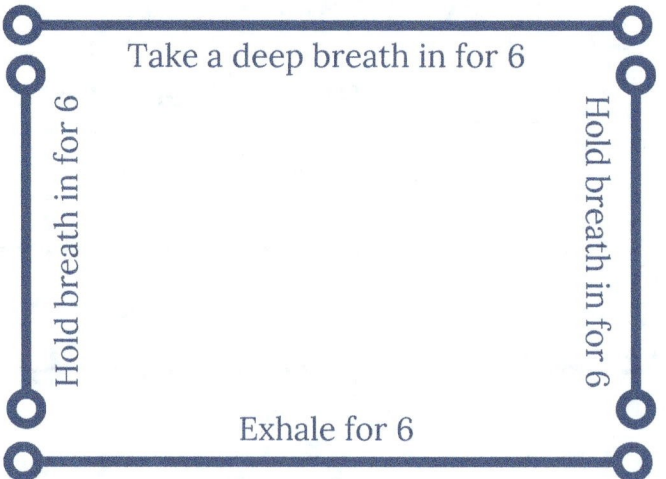

Take a deep breath in for 6

Hold breath in for 6

Hold breath in for 6

Exhale for 6

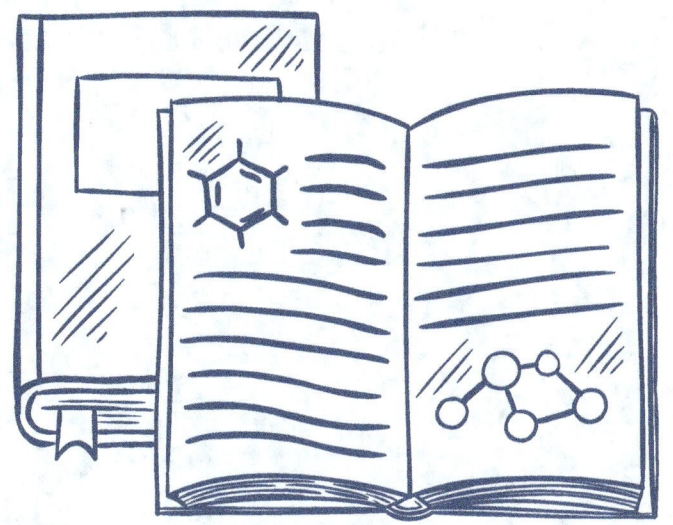

Birth Research

The purpose of Birth Planning is to allow you to research all your options. They allow you to understand backroads incase your journey hits a plot twist. Please take the time to use our light version of a birth plan for your own journey. It can be easily filled out and taken to your provider if you have further questions....

SECRET MENU

VAGINAL SEEDING
A swab to capture the flora to give to baby to help their gut

SKIN TO SKIN
Guaranteed to satisfy you!

DELAYED CORD CLAMPING
Allows for all the goodness from placenta to pass to baby by around 3 minutes after birth

BIRTHER

CLEAR DRAPE
A scrumptious classic, available at most hospitals but a good substitute is having baby peep over drape.

ESSENTIAL OILS & MUSIC
Double comfort measures for birther that can keep space more tranquil

NODES PLACED ON BACK
This allows for ease of movement and breastfeeding

PHOTOGRAPHY
Memories and honoring the moment with snapshots

SLIENCE
Not hearing the OR staff talk about their kid's soccer practice or upcoming vacation can keep the mood on point

SUPPORT

DOULA IN OR
The perfect sweetness to add to any OR

PARTNER STAYING WITH BABY
Our best-seller! This is an easy request that can fulfilled just about everytime.

BE SURE TO TALK
PROVIDER ABOUT THEIR SECRET MENU

Birth Choices

Birth Name:

Partner:

Provider:

Pediatrician:

Baby Name:

Prior to Birth, I would like

- ☐ to meet with members of the OR team who will be with me during delivery
- ☐ an explanation of the procedure before I am taken to the OR
- ☐ an explanation of the medications that will be used
- ☐ my partner/spouse/family member/doula to accompany me in the delivery room

For Pain Relief, I would like

- ☐ Epidural
- ☐ Spinal
- ☐ General Anesthesia

During Birth, I would like

- ☐ to wear my own labor and delivery gown
- ☐ to choose the music playing in OR
- ☐ ECG leads placed on my back
- ☐ my support to take pictures/video
- ☐ the procedure explained as it happens
- ☐ a clear or lowered drape
- ☐ to have a slow delivery
- ☐ Side Conversation limited
- ☐ No Students

Immediately following Birth, I would like

- ☐ my partner in the OR to announce the gender of our baby
- ☐ to delay cord clamping
- ☐ my spouse/partner to cut the umbilical cord
- ☐ immediate skin-to-skin on me or my partner
- ☐ vaginal seeding to be performed
- ☐ to have measurements/assessments performed while the baby is on my chest if they are needed immediately
- ☐ do not give me sedatives after the birth
- ☐ to see and touch the placenta and cord
- ☐ to have the opportunity to breastfeed in the OR

During Recovery, I would like

- ☐ a lactation consultant to visit
- ☐ my other children to come in to meet the new baby
- ☐ family to visit within 1-3 hours after birth
- ☐ my IV, catheter, ECG leads, etc. removed as soon as possible
- ☐ to eat and get up to use the restroom as soon as I feel ready and able to following delivery
- ☐ Limited interaction with nursing staff in night hours to allow rest and bonding
- ☐ a breast pump accessible in my room

Postpartum

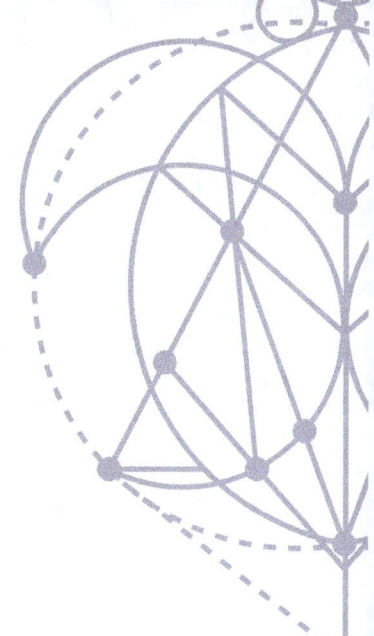

S N O W B A L L

Resources that you'll need

_____

_____

_____

_____

Presenting of your Certificate of Birth Wisdom

DOODLES & NOTES

DOODLES & NOTES

DOODLES & NOTES

DOODLES & NOTES

DOODLES & NOTES

DOODLES & NOTES

DOODLES & NOTES

DOODLES & NOTES

DOODLES & NOTES

DOODLES & NOTES

DOODLES & NOTES

DOODLES & NOTES

DOODLES & NOTES